BIKINI CION

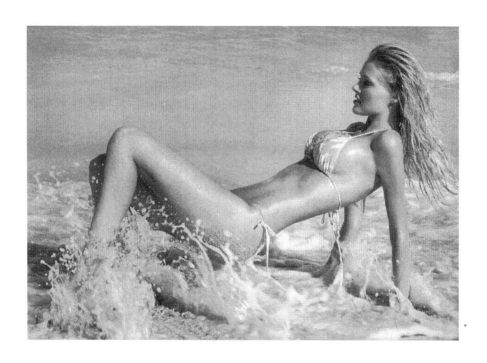

Ultimate Bikini Competition Prep Guide

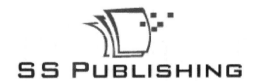

Copyright © 2015 by SS Publishing

All rights reserved. This book or any portion thereof may not be reproduced or used in any manner whatsoever with the express written permission of the publisher except for the use of brief quotations in a book review

Table of Contents

Introduction 1

Chapter 1- Learning about Bikini Competition 3

Chapter 2 – What to look for in a Bikini Coach 9

    Are their services worth it? 9

    So how do you choose your coach if you decide to have one? 10

    What sporting equipment is available? 10

    What moral support will a coach give? 11

    Food and nutritional advice 11

Chapter 3- Ready to Start Training 13

Chapter 4 - Planning Your Meals 23

Chapter 5- Time to Hit the Gym 29

Chapter 6- Catching the Judges Attention with Your Pose 35

    A word of warning 37

Chapter 7 – Body and Hair Preparation 39

    Body hair 39

    The importance of exfoliation 40

    Hair preparation 42

Chapter 8 - Competition Day 45

Conclusion 49

Will You Review My Book? 50

Other Recommendations 51

Introduction

I want to thank you and congratulate you for purchasing the book, *"Ultimate Bikini Competition Prep Guide"*.

This book contains proven steps and strategies ways that you can help to improve your chances of becoming a contestant in a bikini competition. Not only that, you may find that it's the one book that can give you the edge in the contest, covering all of the different aspects that you need to look into to give yourself the best chance possible.

This book not only covers what type of exercises will benefit you the most in training for a bikini competition but also what type of diet plan you should be on. You are also offered tips on when and where you should purchase your bikini during your training process. It also informs you on what will be expected from you during the process of a bikini competition.

With beauty tips and tricks along the way, you will be able to keep this book as your guide during the preparation for the contest, knowing that the information that is contained within the book is written especially for you. We know how important that contest is to you, and with these tips, you will be able to hit all the right buttons with the judges!

Personal beauty tips, posture and pose tips and a lot more than that is all collated in one place. Why? Because I've been there. I've stood on that stage and I know just how frightening it is. I didn't have a guidebook to help me and relied upon my own intuition. Intuition isn't enough. You do need more than that to win, as I found out. This book is my accumulated knowledge put in one easy to read place to help girls going through all of the contest butterflies.

I wish you the best of luck in pursuing your dreams of entering a bikini competition—the main thing to remember is to have fun and enjoy it! Winning is great, but participating also creates great memories and some of the contestants that you meet will be memorable ones that may even become your friends.

CHAPTER 1

Learning About Bikini Competition

When you think about bikinis, you are probably picturing a wonderful time hanging out at the beach on a great sunny summer day! You may also notice the women in bikinis that have amazing shape and muscle tone. This is what is celebrated in a bikini competition. Believe it or not the bikini surfaced during World War II when cloth was being rationed so instead of wearing one-piece bathing suits more women started wearing two-piece bathing suits. From that point on the bikini was here to stay. It was very popular with models, movie stars, and was even featured on the front cover of Playboy in 1962.

During the Festival of Britain in 1951, it is thought that this is where the first bikini competition took place. The contest was named "The Festival Bikini Contest" and was won by a lovely Swedish woman named KiKi Hakanson. Bikini contests really took on in the 80's in the United States, contests such as the Candy Store Bikini Contest, and Miss Midwest Fireworks were very popular. Hawaii and Florida were very popular areas for bikini competitions.

There is another branch of bikini contests that are affiliated with well-known associations such as IFBBF (International Federation of Bodybuilding & Fitness), and the NABBA (National Amateur Body

BIKINI COMPETITION

Building Association). NABBA jumped into the bikini contests in the 80's, IFBBF finally jumped on the bandwagon in 2010. This federation introduced bikini contests that weren't based on muscular builds. For the most part bikini contest are more focused on the female petite shape and form rather than muscular build.

If you are a woman that is happy with the way that you look in your bikini and are interested in competing in some bikini contests then you need to do some research to find out what competitions are going on where and when.

Organizations that Hold Bikini Competitions. A good place to start when trying to find out the pros and cons of the bikini competitions being offered is to try the major federations first. Listed below are a few federations, associations, and organizations that hold bikini competitions regularly.

International Natural Bodybuilding Association—it holds the Bikini Mamas competition, and the annual Bikini Divas competition. Events for the competitions take place in different areas around the country, mainly in the Southwest, in states like California, Arizona, and Texas.

American Natural Bodybuilding Federation—they have bikini division events in group comparisons, and individual presentation, you can find full details of this on their website

Fitness Atlantic—this organization has a diva bikini model section or division

You will be able to check out the different bikini competition that you are interested in competing in. You will be able to find out through the competitions guidelines if it is a competition suited for your body type. Most of these competitions will let you know what kind of body they are looking for whether it is a toned body, or a more muscular type of body.

If you are serious about competing then you are going to have to get some preparations in order for the competition. You are going to have to get into a serious workout routine as well as strict diet plan. It will involve some intense preparation on your part.

Getting a Coach. If you are a beginner in this type of competition you may want to consider getting yourself a coach. It is highly likely that many of those you will be competing against will be coached. You will learn that there is a lot more technique involved in this type of competition than perhaps you were aware of.

Your coach will put you on a specific diet plan and training regimen; your coach will also share with you her knowledge of how the judges work. It is important to choose a coach that has experience with bikini competitions. Do some research on the Internet to find a coach that has good reviews and more importantly a good track record. There are bikini competition coaches that have long track records and highly developed methods of training.

To get a full listing of bikini contests from the Internet for your area and keep up to date with news on events that may be of interest to you. As you need preparation for these events, you also need to ask a coach if they feel that you would qualify for the event that you have in mind.

BIKINI COMPETITION

Remember, there are different types of bikini contest. Some will be where the contestants are judged on beauty, stance and confidence whereas others lean more toward physical fitness or muscle development. You need to decide early on which kind of contest it is that you want to enter as those which are based on weight training will require a lot of training in advance because many of the other contestants will be accustomed to this type of contest and may be tough to beat. However, if you believe you have the looks, the figure and the physique, then now's the time to make the most of it all and get into training.

You will also need to register your interest or have your trainer register you for the bikini contest. The coach is likely to help you to get through all the hassle of registering and preparing and if you are thinking of joining the International circuit, then you need to get everything in place fairly rapidly because you will also have travel arrangements to make to get to the contests in other countries. Canada, the United Kingdom, Africa, Asia and Australia are all contests that you may be interested in qualifying for so the sooner you get information, the better.

If you have already been in a contest and want to further your career, there are valuable resources available for models who enter contests like the Natural Bodybuilding contests such as help with choreography, fitness workshops, exercise camps and resources to help you to choose the suitable music to go with your routine. This is more on the professional level and if you need that kind of backup, resources can be found on Natural Body Building Events.com

The more research you do into the various types of contests, the more likely you are to get into a contest that suits your needs or your body type. These are vast events and are worldwide. If you are in the United States, there are also statewide events that you can get involved in and learn the tricks of the bikini contest circuit.

Contact numbers are vital and here are a few which may help you in your search for the right contest and to get hold of dates and all relevant rules. If you have tentative inquiries about the pro circuit, then an email to NaturalBodybuildingEvents@yahoo.com will get you the results that you need. A trainer will also have a list of events and will be able to give you more details.

Once you have expressed an interest in a contest, then contacting the organizers will be something that your trainer will be able to go through with you. It is important to have venue dates, contest rules and to register your interest as soon as you can so you are kept up to date with any changes that happen as well as news on where you will stay during the event.

There's a whole world of competition out there waiting for you. Learn which contests are the best for you and which will help your career, because some of these contests really are a step in the right direction toward modeling and you may just get noticed even if you don't win the contest!

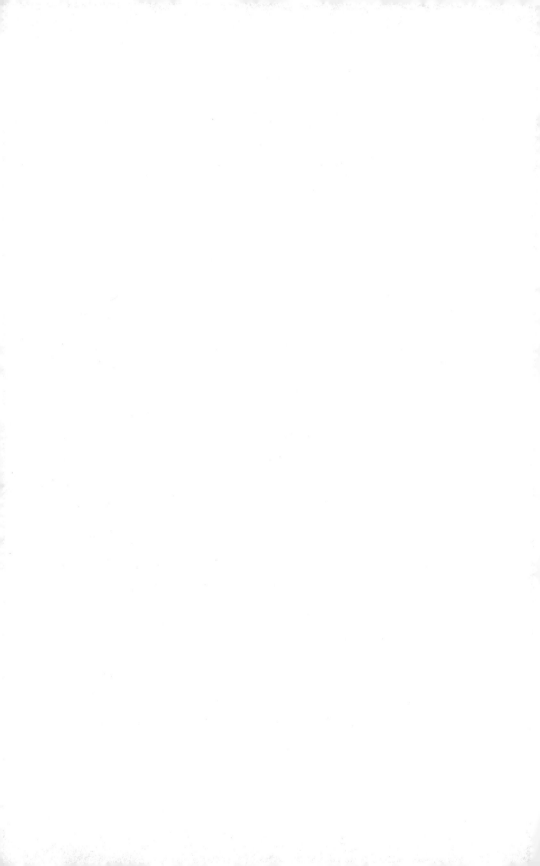

CHAPTER 2

What to look for in a Bikini Coach

The kind of coach that you are looking for depends upon the type of contest that you are considering. If it's simply a bikini contest where the contestants are judged for beauty and grace, you will need a coach that can walk you through your paces. The way that you walk, the way that you stand, the poses that you take all have special significance with the judges and these are the people with a proven track record in the field in which you want to compete.

Are their services worth it?

It really depends upon how much you want to win. Many trainers will be proud to show you how high their hit rate is and how the contestants that they prep get into the first three positions on a regular basis. The services they give you are a complete range of nutritional tips, exercises in posture and walking, shaping up and getting your body ready for the contest.

It's worth it if you think that you want to take the competition seriously. If, however, you want to enter for the fun of it and don't really care about your placement, then perhaps reading up on all the aspects is sufficient for you. It may actually be your natural charm that wins the day, but it's unlikely. These ladies that take on the bikini world and train contestants know what they are doing.

So how do you choose your coach if you decide to have one?

The first thing you need to know is if they specialize in the kind of contest you have your eye on. For example, is it a contest where you will be judged on your muscle structure and more weight training orientated? If so, then a beauty prep service isn't the right one for you. Meet your coach in person and see whether you also think that your personalities will complement each other. It's hard to take advice from someone that you don't really get on with. Some coaches will give you the impression that they are trying to live up to their unrealized dreams by putting others through their paces. They may be pushy and have personalities that you find too strong to work with.

Others will understand all of the intricacies of what it means to walk down that catwalk showing your skin to the whole world and making a mess of it. They've seen the heartbreak. They have been there to watch their models get through their paces. See if the coach is empathetic because if she can put herself in your shoes, chances are that she will be understanding and agreeable to get on with.

What sporting equipment is available?

You may need to know this, especially if you are entering a contest where you will be judged solely on the presentation of your body. If there is a gym, is there qualified staff to help you out in weak areas?

What moral support will a coach give?

For the purpose of finding out whether a coach is suitable, read testimonials. See images of their successful models because a picture can tell you a lot about the model's chances of success and testimonials tell you what the model thought of the service being offered.

Food and nutritional advice

An all in service should give you nutritional advice that will help you to present yourself in a really healthy looking way. It's not just about diet. It's about shining hair, soft skin and caring for yourself so that it shows when you walk down the catwalk. Check into what is on offer and don't take anyone's word for it. You are paying for this service. If you really want to win badly enough, you will want to know what your chances are and what the coaching service can do for you.

Don't take it for granted that online coaches give you the same attention as offline ones. There may be a price differential between online and offline training, but look at the whole package and see what you are getting for your money. For example, a fully backed online coaching service may set you back a one time fee of about $300 or as much as $200 a month. Are you prepared to make an investment of that kind? Only you can decide if this is a career move or if it's merely wanting to measure yourself against other competitors.

The last thing to look out for is to see what facilities a coach has to put you in touch with the right people for your final presentation. Skin presentation and waxing will be necessary before the contest and you may want to take advantage of getting your body bronzed beforehand. A good coach will know what services are available and will be able to put you in touch with the right people and that's going to be a lot better than hit and miss contacts. Trust your coach.

You need to have a coach with the kind of character that can push you to get the best out of you. You also need him/her to be someone you really do feel you can work with.

A wrong choice could mean losing the game before you have even started. Their personality has to fit with yours. Sure, they are going to be tough but you are probably a tough cookie to crack anyway, and toughness may be exactly what you need to get you in shape ready for the contest.

You must know exactly what services are included in the package when you sign up and you should make sure that you are aware of what the price you pay includes and for how long. Support right up to the contest date is best because that means that your coach sticks with it and will be there to advise at the last minute and that could be essential.

There are various packages available over the Internet but don't be too quick to jump in and take the first one that comes up. It's far better to have a personal trainer who you can meet on a regular basis and who will help you to get through the preparation than to have one at a distance that you can never get hold of when you need to. You also need to compare prices and what you get for your money because this is vital to your success.

CHAPTER 3

Ready to Start Training

You should think about spending at least twelve weeks in training before the competition. You are probably in fairly good shape at this point since you are keen on entering a bikini contest. You are probably at a decent weight now, with a modest amount of body fat but you do need to keep an eye on it and maximize your potential to win the contest. It could mean a modeling contract and send your career in the right direction. If you are going in for a hot competition which calls for muscle development, you may need longer to prepare for your contest and it would be a good idea to consult in person with a coach so that they can establish your body shape and the amount of work that you need to get you in shape for the contest. You can't generalize about a thing like this on the pro circuit because your competition is very tough and your coach will know when she/he meets you exactly what training you need.

Week 1

1. Make sure to do your research and get yourself mentally prepared for your intense training that lies just ahead. Try and hire a coach by the end of this week if you haven't done so yet. A coach can mean the world of difference to your preparation and to your ultimate success. Use the criteria explained in the last chapter and do compare what each coach you consider has on offer and what their track record is.

2. Do your research into the proper diet and study and learn how macronutrients, fats, and carbs all affect your body. Your coach will help you with this but you should be in control and do your own research and educate yourself on proper diet plans. Diet plans must also take into account the effects of bloating, as these can be disastrous on the contest day. Coaches who are experienced will know all the answers to help you to avoid such a disaster and will pass all their secrets on to you. If you choose to train without a coach, then do look into the effects that your food has on you and avoid foods that will cause bloat especially in the days that lead to the competition heats.

3. Start to plan your workouts and diet plan with your coach. If you haven't got a coach yet start making plans on your own. But if you are really serious about doing well in these competitions and want to get noticed then you should hire a coach to guide you on the best things needed from you in order to win at a bikini competition. By the end of week one, you should have a good idea of what you are not permitted to eat and what foods are actually useful to you. There are certain foods that help to promote shiny hair and these may be useful to you. The coaches know all the tricks but that doesn't mean you can't find out a few of your own on the way.

4. Tell your friends and family of your plans this will help to setup a support system for you. Explain that you will be on a strict diet to get yourself in shape for the competition, ask them to help you in this area by not stopping by with a box of doughnuts for example. But instead, they will be able to help to give you that support you are going to need during this process to keep you motivated and positive that you can

do this. They may even want to chip in a little on the cost of a coach!

At this stage of the game, it's a good idea to use Google Images to find the image you think is your ideal of how a bikini should be presented. If you type in a search into Google Images using the keywords Bikini contest, you will get a great idea about what you are aiming for. Look which color bikini goes well with your hair color as there are pages and pages of photographs of past contests which will show you all the victories but also give you an idea of what to avoid. This is important during this week because this will show you what you want to look like. The bikinis in different colors and also with different shapes of tops will give you a great idea about which suits your breast shape. Look for other women with similar size to you and see how they presented themselves because it will show you errors in judgment and it will also show you many ideas that worked.

Use this exercise for example to show you how people have been able to hide flaws or to see what the difference poses are because you need to see the whole picture. You – the bikini – the pose – the colors – the bling. Then you need to look at the makeup, the hairstyles and the tattoos. Judges may not be too keen on them but it's quite a common thing these days. What I found from looking at bikini contest images was what not to do. Some girls had used too much body oil and although it looked fairly cool, they had managed to get it into their hair, so that the ends of their hair looked greasy. Others had used just the right amount and their skin looked really fresh and clean, young and healthy. Yet others chose not to use oils and looked a little dried out in comparison.

Why this on week one? There's a very good reason. If you know what you are heading for then you can try out all the products and get yourself prepared well in advance of the contest. There's no last minute mistake. That's very important indeed. The pictures helped me to find the image that I wanted people to see when they looked at me in my bikini. When I found the perfect look, I then geared my training around achieving it.

Week 2

1. You will begin your workout regimen with the help and guidance of your coach. You will be given further details of a good regimen in chapter 4. Try not to cheat as you will only be cheating yourself and that's not what it's all about. Remember, the sooner you fix a regime, the sooner you will find it comes as second nature and you know that your win depends upon you being sensible about the training. If you're not serious about it, how can you expect to win?

2. It is also time to begin your diet regimen. At this time, you will be focusing on a diet that will help you in supporting your muscle growth and most importantly supporting good health. You will find the diet in more detail in chapter 3. People tend to be a little lethargic when it comes to keeping to a dietary routine. However, you have a goal in mind and you won't get there unless you are prepared to work for it. You may think yourself slim and lovely, but it's not about slimming. It's about getting your body toned to perfection because judges are going to be looking for the best tone, rather than the prettiest face.

3. You need to make hair and beauty appointments for the morning

of your competition. You may think this is too early, but it is better to get these things taken care of so that you are not running around at the last minute trying to find a beauty salon that can fit you in. You will already be feeling stressed on the day of the competition you don't want to worry about things that you don't have to. It is much better to be prepared early than to leave it until it is too late. I have a tip here that helped me considerably. If you are going to have your hair cut do it weeks in advance and just get a trim on the day. That way, you won't have to contend with hair is unpredictable and will be accustomed to the style chosen. Often people lose confidence when they have a haircut or a change of style until they are accustomed to it. The last thing that you want on the day before the contest is a change you were not prepared for.

4. Ask a friend or family member to be your moral support during the eleven weeks that you will be training and dieting. Tell your social group what is going on so they are all in the loop at what you need during that eleven weeks. You may have to avoid certain social events so that you are not tempted to waver off your strict diet regimen. Letting everyone know what is going on will help to keep your morale up. The more support you have the better your chances of success are. Think of these people as being your cheerleaders.

Week 3

1. At this point you will be stepping up the workout, with the guidance of your coach. Do take notice. Your coach knows what is best for your body and how much you can take. Remember that you are nearing the contest and that all this training will pay off. Keep your mind focused

on winning and make sure that you go the extra mile with your training. Never take shortcuts and don't think that the coach won't notice if you miss out on a few exercises. It's only you that wants to win this contest and you will be kidding yourself if you think you can wing it without putting in the hard work. There are others out there that will and they will come off better in competition if you don't pull your weight.

2. You will be deep into your diet regimen at this point, keeping your support system close at hand to help coax you through those weak moments.

You can also step these up in different directions if you find that you need to. For example, if your food is giving you bloat, learn to drink lots of water and to adjust the times that you eat to fit with your exercise routine. Remember to take notes because bloat at the wrong moment during a contest won't do you any favors. Thus write down what you ate, and at what time followed by whether it bloated your stomach or not, as on the day of the contest, you have to be sure that the food you eat won't give you the same effect. Even if this is a favorite food, wait until after the contest.

Week 4

1. Your workout regimen is continued and is over-viewed carefully by your coach. As you work out, your coach will observe you, she will then give you tips on how you can improve your workout by changing certain positions or your approach etc. She will show you how to benefit the most from your workout regimen. Your coach is going to also push you to do better and excel in your workout performance,

based on your personal circumstances. For example, you may have great legs but need work on the abs. Only your coach will know and if changes are made to your routine, these will be to solidify your chances of winning and based upon what your coach feels are your weak areas.

2. You will start to observe at this point to see how your calves, and glutes are progressing. This is described in chapter 4. Be proud of your achievements and use this to motivate you to continue.

3. With your diet you will see modest results but you must remember that you are not on some crash diet attempting to lose 30 pounds. You are trying to tone and slim while trying to keep a modest growth of muscles alive and healthy. So don't be discouraged if you haven't lost major weight, instead you should be happy as losing a large amount of weight is not the focus of your diet.

4. This is when you must begin practicing some of the poses you are going to use during the bikini competition. These will be discussed further in chapter 5 but basically this is going to be when you need to make yourself a chart and have a full length mirror at your disposal so that you can practice in your contest shoes and this includes the walk, the turn, taking to steps, going down steps, standing to talk to the judges. You need to be perfect for this and it takes a lot of preparation but this is fun preparation rather than really hard work. It also gives you a chance to see your bikini and how it moves when you move your body. This will also give you clues as to where you need to apply bikini glue. The last thing that you need is for your nipple to expose itself as you turn! It has happened on the stage so don't think this is

a joke. With clothing that is so small, bikini glue may be a lifesaver.

5. Go with a friend or your support system to begin to research bikinis, compare the prices and styles of various stores etc. If you want to have a custom suit made you may have to book this five weeks in advance. So you must make sure you are organized to set this up on time.

If you want to have a bikini made for you then you need to make sure that you are going to have your bikini ready and waiting for you in plenty of time before the competition. Use a store that has a good reputation for getting items complete on time and for guaranteeing good quality work. It may also be a good idea to watch the kind of bikinis that are being used for these contests in recent events, because you want to look outstanding and will want to test that the bikini fits in all the right places. An off the shelf bikini may not be good enough to get you noticed from the crowd. Always abide by the rules of the contest and don't go mini when you are not supposed to. These are bikini contests, not porn shows and you may be disqualified if you try to look too risqué.

Week 5

1. You continue to do your workout under the guidance of your coach, and stick to your strict diet regimen.

2. It is time to go shoe shopping for a pair of high heels that you will be wearing in the competition. Bring a friend or your support system along it always helps when you have a second opinion when you are unsure. Once you have your new heels you must begin to practice

posing and walking in them. You want to know how to turn in your heels going from one stance to another in a free flowing manner.

Week 6-8

1. You need to get your poses down then begin to practice just like you are in a real competition. You need to get yourself to a point that it feels natural to you.

2. It is important that you stay focused at this point as you are now past the halfway point to reaching your goal! Your workout is very hard and demanding and so is your diet regimen, but you are going to benefit immensely from them. To make yourself feel better you should look at photos of yourself before you began to train, you will see positive results at this point that will certainly cheer you up.

Week 9

1. You need to start getting the jewelry together that you are planning to wear for the bikini competition. Lay out the different pieces of jewelry that you have chosen and ask your friend's opinion on the pieces they think suit you the best. You may have to go out and buy some new jewelry for this competition but it doesn't have to be that expensive. As long as it complements the bikini and helps in your overall presentation, that's good enough.

2. Get yourself organized by getting all of your supplies together and ready for the competition. Work on getting yourself mentally prepared for the competition that will be full of surprises, excitement, and nervousness.

Week 10

1. You should have your poses down at this point. You should add some twists at certain points to give some sass to your poses.

2. Maintaining your weight and your protein is important at this point in the diet. Just try and avoid cheating!

Week 11

1. Get the bikini wax done and make sure to have your entire body shaved or have hair removal. It's always better if you keep hair removal as a top priority and keep your skin exfoliated because you will need to use tanning products and these really don't do well on skin that is stubbly.

2. Get a small audience of friends to do a practice walk for. This will help you to get used to doing your routine in front of people. If you could do some practice sessions perhaps at local school auditorium that has a stage, then have your viewers below you like the judges will be in competition.

Week 12

This is time to get you prepared to travel to the location the competition is being held.

1. Make sure to do a last body shave before you leave for competition.

2. Pack all of your supplies the night before so you are ready to go on the day of competition.

CHAPTER 4

Planning Your Meals

When you are up on the stage during the competition strutting across it giving it your all with every twist, turn and pose, it will not be your hot body that will win this for you but your brain. Using your brains gray matter, you were able to understand the importance of a healthy regimen that includes balanced nutrition, elimination of certain foods, and exercise, and also the self-control that was needed for you to get to the competition was crucial.

Eating Clean

The phrase "eating clean" is a very common one in the fitness training world. For many, this means being able to pack as many nutrients into their low calorie count as possible. Some of the foods that are known as staples in the eating clean system for a bikini competitions are:

Lean meats—meats that have a high fat content are not allowed for the 12 weeks of intense dieting for competition. You must choose instead thin turkey slices, or chicken, fish such as cod, whitefish or tilapia. These are lean meats that will provide you with good healthy protein to help support your muscle development. That may not seem a huge issue for you but it is vital that you have your share of this kind of protein so don't merely cut out red meat. Replace it with white meat because it helps you to develop the shape that will be ideal for displaying your body.

Complex carbs and simple carbs are pretty much off the menu during training period and this includes anything that is not labeled 100% whole grain. Whole grains help to stop your blood sugar from leaping up and down all over the place. You can't afford to have an unpredictable diet at this stage of the game if you want to win the contest.

Select vegetables—but because there are vegetables that have a high glycemic content they are off the menu such as potatoes, starchy veggies like carrots and turnips, which should only be used in moderation. Veggies that are good choices are squash, cauliflower, broccoli and green beans. These will roast really nicely to give you a caramelized taste without making them taste boring.

Secret Food Weapons

Here are a few food items that you may not be aware of that can be helpful during your diet regimen.

Stevia—this is an all-natural sweetener and is calorie-free. You can mix it in with Greek yogurt to make yourself a nice pudding. Add some cocoa or lemon to it to add to the flavor.

Buckwheat Flour—this is not a type of wheat. It is gluten-free fruit seed that is related to rhubarb. You can use this flour to make muffins, scones, or pancakes. You can use these in a great breakfast for yourself. Just don't be eating them throughout the day—everything in moderation.

Avocado-this is great to add on top of some rice or as part of a salad. This is a healthy source of fat that can enhance your snacks and salads as well as leave you feeling great because the cholesterol they provide is good cholesterol and helps to keep your circulation in a fit state.

Casein—this is a protein it is the main ingredient found in cheese. You can also buy puddings, and shakes that are made with it. You can use this to allow yourself to have a sweet treat that is low-calorie and supplies you with protein.

Twelve Weeks

There are various ways that you can plan your diet and the best thing to do is to discuss this with your coach and see what she suggests to be a good choice. After all, she is the one that is experienced in these areas, and you are relying on her experience to help you make the best choices so that you may succeed in your goals. Remember that you are paying for her advice, so you are defeating the object if you ignore it.

Carb Cycling

Carb cycling is referring to when people that are in training will have days in their training period with "high carb days" and "no-carb or low-carb days." The idea behind this is to limit carbs on some days, then switch to having carbs on other days so that you are not starving your body of carbs.

Remember to keep in mind on the days that you are getting carbs this does not mean pigging out on foods like waffles and syrup. What you are trying to do on these days is to give yourself enough energy so that you are not starving your body of carbs.

You and your coach may decide not to put you on a cycling program—but instead, focus more on the portion sizes, low calories, and healthy ingredients in your diet. The decision whether to put you on a cycle program will largely depend on how you feel after each workout. You may decide that you need some heavy carbs after certain workout days.

The main thing you must remember is to limit your calorie intake in carbs. You want to make sure that all or most of the calories you are taking in are packed full of nutrients. Below is an example of a simple meal plan for midway through the program.

Meal 1: Several blueberries, one-third cup of casein pudding, handful of cashews or almonds.

Meal 2: Brown rice cake topped with diced red bell peppers, red onion, avocado slices, and arugula. You could make an avocado spread instead using a food processor, season with dash of lemon, paprika, and one third cup of kidney beans, seasoned with ginger.

Meal 3: One-third cup of tuna stored in water if canned. Add white balsamic vinegar, seasoned with oregano, basil, and garlic powder, diced red onions, diced red bell peppers, serve on brown rice cake, or on lettuce leaf, or one buckwheat and almond scone.

Meal 4: 2-3 ounces of thinly sliced turkey breast with a moderate amount of avocado spread or with mustard, one third cup of sautéed kale or spinach, almond slivers, diced red onion, one third cup of

Greek yogurt with some Stevia and cocoa.

Just because you are eating low-calorie foods does not mean they have no flavor. You can season your foods with things such as ginger, fresh herbs, bell peppers, and red onions. Learn how to flavor your quinoa, or rice with Asian flavors. Also use these to flavor your chicken, fish, and turkey. You will enjoy your meals when adding some fun flavors to them rather than feeling like you are being deprived of flavorful meals.

Don't beat yourself up if you occasionally do have something that you shouldn't but be very aware of what foods bloat you because these are not the foods to eat near to the contest. The last thing that you want is for your stomach to look huge and some foods can even bloat the upper abdomen so avoid them if you notice any bloat whatsoever.

The most important thing to think about is drinking water and lots of it during training. If you can adapt this habit in your general lifestyle, you will find that it improves skin elasticity, helps your hair to look healthy and really does help the body to feel supple and young. I know water is boring. I've been there and felt the same way as you do, but I have actually benefited from drinking water because my skin stayed young looking as compared with my sister's skin, which is badly wrinkled. There is more than just skin care involved. Hydration of the body's organs and the inner workings is vital. If you have to, space your drinks but do put out sufficient in the mornings, so you can always carry a bottle with you.

CHAPTER 5

Time to Hit the Gym

During your training period of twelve weeks you are going to be involved in some High Intensity Interval Training (HIIT). High Intensity Interval Training is the best approach for a short program such as yours. It is based around working very hard for quick intervals, 20-30 seconds, with rest periods of less strenuous work such as walking. During each burst there is a wide variety of exercises, such as sprints, squats, rowing machine, thrusts, push-ups, knee-bends, etc.

When you blast into quick intense bursts of activity this causes your body to need large amounts of oxygen. During the recovery, your body is in a state of oxygen shortage, and will burn more fat. Thus, it works to keep you in shape.

Your coach may be familiar with many different HIIT regimens. She will guide you to the areas that need to be HIIT.

Glutes—in the bikini contest your glutes are indeed a big area that is focused on during the competition. There are competitions that will give you tips on how they want you to round out the booty and how it should be framed in your bikini.

These are some sample workouts you can do for glutes:

Do each exercise for 30 seconds then rest for 10 seconds before the next burst.

BIKINI COMPETITION

1. Jump squats

2. Half burpee with dead lift use a kettle ball that weights between 15-20 pounds

3. Jump rope

4. Break-dancer planks

Here is Gym Version:

These exercises are using weight machines:

1. Using leg press, do three sets of 12-18, progressing during your plan.

2. Wall squat with a stability ball, place ball between you and the wall and do three sets of 12-18 per leg.

3. Leg-press kickbacks do three sets of 12-18.

Hamstrings workout. The hamstrings are the muscles at the top and back of your legs. These are important to get them looking at their best especially during a bikini competition.

Do the following exercises for 30 seconds and 20 seconds between each exercise.

1. Fire hydrant—gym version

2. Donkey kicks—each side

3. Kettle ball swing 10-15 pounds

BIKINI COMPETITION

Gym Version:

1. Seated hamstring curl (leg curl) do four sets 10-15.

2. Lying down leg curls do three sets of 10-15

3. Barbell hip thrust three sets 15-20

Abs workout. Your abs are the third area where much focus will be during the bikini competition. You are going to have to hit your abs pretty hard during the program whether you are looking for washboard abs or just a nice hard tummy.

1. Decline sit-ups three sets of 15

2. Seated knee-ups start with 10-pound kettle ball and progress.

3. Cable bends three sets of 15

Your trainer will be able to give you full details of the kinds of exercises that are known to help you in your presentation. These are people who know all the tricks and will have a proven track record in preparing ladies to look their best on the day of the competition.

Try to take what they say seriously. I know it's hard when you are being pressured into exercise, but it's your idea to be in the contest and the exercises are simply a consequence of YOUR choice. You can go into a contest half=heartedly, but it's unlikely that you will win if you do. Thus, taking your trainer seriously really will help you.

Your body is exposed to all kinds of pressure in the gym. It's important that you sleep for sufficient hours to let any injured part of your body heal naturally during sleep. This is also important for your looks. If you overwork yourself and cut out sufficient sleep, it will look like you did just that when you hit the contest line up.

If the kind of contest that you are entering is one based on muscle formation, then you may have to work a little harder to get in shape and to help develop the muscles so that they look great on the day. One point to remember is that when you subject yourself to a heavy exercise routine and then stop between contests, what you leave yourself open to is weight gain and flab. It is wise to keep up the exercise and diet routine even after the contest is over. You can be a little more lax but if you intend to enter more contests, don't make it harder work than you have to by lapsing into old habits between contests. The yoyo effect on your body can be very detrimental.

Making exercise fun as well

It's important that you have fun with exercise as well to keep you in trim. Aside from the obvious exercises, dancing or Zumba can be really good fun and can help you to exercise all the different parts of the body in a fun routine that energizes you. Make sure that you drink sufficient water, but believe me, this kind of exercise in between standard exercises really does help you because the mobility of your body and the way that it works your legs, arms and every other part of the body can make your general routine exercises easier to bear.

Remember, you are in this because you want to be. Having a little fun in between time which provides great exercise really will help you to keep your motivation going and show your friends that you really are serious about your competitiveness.

Talk to your trainer about what you can do in between exercise sessions, as they may encourage fun activities such as swimming or other sports within your area that are going to be enjoyable. Team sports such as tennis are good because these help mobility and help you to keep your body in trim, but they do more than that. If you are competing with someone else, you won't let him or her down by not turning up. Thus, if you have a friend that is supporting your exercise regime, this friend is the perfect ally for a swimming outing or a game of tennis on a friendly basis to take the work out of the exercise part of your preparation.

CHAPTER 6

Catching the Judges Attention with Your Pose

It is very important during a competition that you pose correctly as you are not only judged on looks. You are going to be judged on the technique that you use to strike poses and show yourself in the proper form. As I mentioned in chapter 3 you need to have started practicing your poses in week four of your twelve-week training period.

You may be wondering why you have to start learning your poses this early in your training. The reason is that you want to have time to practice your routine wearing your high heels to the point that you know every move inside out. So during the competition if you become a bit nervous you can still do your poses with no problems. The poses you need to learn are the following:

1. Front Stances. This is when you are at center stage giving the judges a front view of yourself and smiling at them. Make sure that you have your feet almost shoulder-width, straight but not rigid. There are competitors that choose to place one hand on the hip at this point then alternate. You need a pose that looks natural and not overdone. Remember that you are what the judges are looking at and this front stance can make or break your potential to win. Practice it using a full-length mirror and practice it some more because anything can happen.

BIKINI COMPETITION

Check out your smile before you hit the stage. The last thing you need is a little bit of salad left on your teeth from lunch!

2. 180 degree turn. You are moving your position so that you will end up with your back to the judges. Halfway through this move you are expected to shoot the judges a smile. Make sure to have the timing down on this. Give a long look and smile over your shoulder. This may sound straightforward but it's not as easy as you think, bearing in mind you have new high heeled shoes on and are walking on an unfamiliar surface.

3. Back Stance. Once you are in your back stance position you are going to show off your glutes and hammies by slightly leaning forward. Doing this move will get rid of the crease in the middle of your bikini. You may choose to cross your legs during this stance and this will be up to you and your coach. Remember, the judges have to judge you on all of these poses as well as upon their initial impression of you. Look at winners on Google Images and you can pretty well gage what it is that they are looking for.

These are the mandatory poses that you will have to do in major bikini competitions. You are given a little personal flexibility in how you perform them but basically, you do need to include them in your routine to abide by the contest rules.

The walk out center stage is also very important accompanied by your music showing the judges what you look like in motion. You should try and walk with firm confident steps much in the same manner as a runway model. You may choose not to smile through the walk, since this could appear to be unnatural or a little preconceived. You could give a poised and determined look then soften it up when you are getting into your poses.

Attitude. This is important to showing the judges that you are able to be fun and serious - showing them that you are not arrogant but are confident and able to have some fun. Judges like to see a popular winner and those who get the art of getting the poses right is likely to be very popular indeed. The right amount of smile, the flow of movement, and the confidence with the poses is all part of what the contest is all about. Don't overdo it because even though you may think you are being clever, the judges can see right through these tactics and are not going to give you extra points because you showed them your teeth over an extended period of time. They want overall beauty and people don't walk around with a cheesy grin on their faces. It doesn't look natural and isn't the image they are seeking.

Practice the walk, the turn, the bend, the smiles and the twists because on stage you don't get a second chance. Make sure the shoes you practice in are the shoes you will wear for the contest and be proud as you stride across the stage gracefully in them. It takes practice. You can have the most beautiful body on the stage but if you can't walk in those heels, you are not going to create the right impression with the judges.

A word of warning

You do need to practice with your shoes on. It's absolutely essential and it's also important that you practice all poses with the shoes on different types of surface so that you gain absolute confidence. You also need to walk up and down steps to gain confidence if faced with hurdles such as this. Bear in mind that if you use any lotion on your body, your feet are likely to feel slippery in your shoes. Practice with the same body cream that you will use when you compete because otherwise you may find it's an absolute disaster. Grip of your feet inside those shoes is essential. Thus remember the use of body oils because this may catch you out if you are not prepared.

CHAPTER 7

Body and Hair Preparation

While we have talked about this briefly, you need to be aware of what it takes to get your body looking great. This means every inch of you because if there's something wrong, someone will notice it.

Body hair

Although you may be accustomed to body hair removal, it's not a good idea to shave. If you can use creams, you are much less likely to create stubble that someone will notice. Plus, creams last longer and are gentler on your skin than a razor. Imagine getting a shaving rash on the day of the contest! It does happen if you are not gentle with your skin. Remember that your bikini line and any facial hair will need to be dealt with by a beautician. This isn't an expensive process but if you can arrange it as near to the contest as possible, it's unlikely that you will have any growth between the beauty treatment and your lineup on the stage.

Underarms must be completely free of hair and if you have dark hair, don't count on a shaver for this area because it will leave stubble that can look very unsightly. Ask your beautician by all means but a good quality cream remover is the best. Just don't do it on the morning of the contest in case this shows redness after the treatment is done.

The importance of exfoliation

The reason you need to exfoliate is so that your skin looks absolutely perfect on the day and can take an even tanning. Dead skin makes your skin look dry and uncared for and that's the last thing you want on that stage, especially if it is a stage that has lighting. Many contestants have said that even with a reasonable tan, your body can look pasty on the stage if you don't prep it and have at least two coats of tanning product.

Start this process early because once you start to use tanning products you can't shave anymore because it is likely that this will affect the tan that you have. Exfoliation is preparation for tanning.

Tanning – Products? Sun Spray Tan? Sun Bed?

The choice is yours though most contestants say that you really do need to present your body with a great tan and this will be a build-up process. I would suggest taking natural tan as far as you can, followed by salon tan because you need the depth of color to actually show up all the surface of your muscles. If you are going for a spray tan, you need your skin to be absolutely clean before it is used. Deodorants and beauty products get in the way and actually can make your skin appear patchy. I take a very baggy tee shirt with me to the salon and make sure that after being sprayed, I don't wear anything that may rub the finish.

Your skin should always be prepped for the tanning and your coach should be able to tell you all the tips and tricks that you can use. Some other girls may have tips to pass on as well.

You need to have all your makeup sorted out so that you have everything that you need with you. Your skin needs to be prepped on the day and if you are wearing false lashes, you need to ensure that you have plenty of prep time before the actual contest, so that you can check yourself over and make sure that you really have prepared for the contest.

I always take someone with me to help me with all the last minute details. How you present your skin is important. The point is though that by the time I get to a contest, I have already done my makeup and it's only last minute touches that need to be done. Oils on the skin are important but whatever you do, don't forget latex gloves to apply this with because your skin and your hands are important and you may end up with discolored hands which is something that the judges are going to notice.

Don't forget your bikini glue. Some of the worst mistakes I have ever seen have been because models forgot to use this essential product. It's not like you are walking across a beach and no one will notice. When you are on the stage, everyone notices, so having your glue available is extremely important. "It Stays" is a pretty cool product and it washes off easily after the contest without having to resort to really strong detergent! If you don't know how to use it, ask your coach.

What this does is keep your bikini in place so that there are no slip-ups when you are on the stage. If you think it's not important, go to an amateur bikini show and look at the rear end of the models. You will see the bikini slipping around all over the place and that's something a judge will most certainly find distracting. Be sure to have this with you on the day. It may just give you the extra confidence that you need.

Hair preparation

You will really want to have your hair sorted out well before the contest. The idea is that a contestant should look naturally beautiful and thus many contests disallow hair accessories. It isn't about pulling your hair back from your face at all. It's a case of letting it hang down and look pretty. You can use jewelry but certainly not anything in your hair, so don't even be tempted to go there or you may find yourself being asked to take accessories out of your hair, messing up your whole idea if you rely upon them.

Your hair should be given more body than usual because you will be judged on it as the premise of the contest is overall beauty of presentation and that means adhering to the rules. There may also be unwritten rules, so make sure that you make yourself aware of everything you are expected to adhere to.

Your hair is your crowning glory and what you look like on the day really does matter. Use products that you trust and don't leave anything to chance. You will be competing with girls that have done this before.

Make-up

There are differing views when it comes to makeup preparation. Some experts say that the eye makeup is the most important, while others say that the emphasis of the facial structure is much more important and that this can be highlighted by correct use of makeup that shows off the cheekbones.

It really depends upon you how far you want to go with your makeup order of priorities, but if people tell you that your eyes are amazing, then you'd be a little neglectful if you didn't do the best that you can to highlight the eyes. Lips that are too full look awful, so avoid that look altogether. The pouting look is so out of date and as you are going for a natural look, the judges are more likely to choose someone who goes for a youthful look rather than that of a vamp.

Nail Prep for Contests

Often people question choices used for contests, but I really think that the focus of attention of the judges should be toward the bikini and body and if you go too flash with your nails, you tend to distract the judges eye and that's not the best way to go. You can choose a French polish style but I tend to use varnishes which are fairly neutral but which show that I actually took care of my finger nails and toe nails. Avoid dark colors like the plague because they look cheap and tacky and in the light of the stage really will draw attention in all the wrong ways.

Lots of girls use bling on toenails just for fun and that's okay but make sure it's not dark because it looks so terrible. If you do go for a French manicure, make sure that you go to someone who knows how to do it correctly because some versions there is such a start contrast between your tips and the actual nail that they look cheap and tacky.

BIKINI COMPETITION

Another place you can look for ideas for your nails is on a website called Pinterest and there are some stunning nail designs which are in pastel shades so they look gorgeous without looking garish and show the judges that you take care of yourself and take a pride in what you look like. Pastel shades are wonderful because they don't give that vamp impression and are pretty and look natural rather than trying to take on the feline look. Some of the designs that you see combine pastel colors and look extremely pretty.

Don't forget also to take extra with you in case your nails get chipped during the prep stages and you need to touch them up ready for the judges.

For your toenails, just go for a color that goes with your overall look without making them the feature when people look at you. It's not about your feet. It's about your overall presentation. If you overdo it, then you can bet your boots that the judges will be looking at your feet and may just be too distracted to notice the great poses that you practiced for hours in front of the mirror. Think subtle. Think pretty and avoid all those nasty tacky reds and will certainly not do you any favors.

CHAPTER 8

Competition Day

Now is the time to congratulate yourself on successfully completing the training by using a lot of self-discipline. You have managed to lose weight and get yourself incredibly toned. Let us talk about getting your supplies ready, and the big day you have worked so hard to get to. You need to hype yourself up but you also need to remain pleasant to other contestants. You are not here to make enemies and the attitude of people who have this selfish need to be best really does show through. Both the judges and the audience can spot a fake a mile away, so be pleasant and be part of the contest, rather than just being there to win.

The Bikini. When it comes to competition-grade bikinis they are made so that they fit your measurements, they are not just any old bikini of the rack. You should be thinking of your suit around the sixth week of your training. You want to get the measurements as close to what you will be during the competition. You do not want to order your bikini in the first week.

Make sure that the store you are getting your bikini done at understands when you need the bikini done by. I always insist on a fitting and a final adjustment if needed, so be careful who you use for your bikini as this can make all the difference in the world to the presentation.

Contests do allow off the rack bikinis, although you are unlikely to want to use one if you want to make the most of your body for the contest. Made to measure really is the only way to go as the rules insist that your costume is decent and that you have to keep within set guidelines. Make sure you do because being disqualified for something like this could be embarrassing. Also make sure that you get some bikini glue at this stage and are instructed on how best to use it. The last thing you want is for your bikini to give the impression that you are sweating in unladylike places, so get it right. The glue is only used to hold the pieces of the bikini in place in areas where there may be slippage.

Jewelry/ Accessories. These are something you can shop for at any time during the training period that best suits you. Having some bling will help you to look like you are on stage and not just hanging out at the beach. You should look at websites that specialize in competition gear and certainly make sure that it's going to be there on time for the contest. Make sure that you try it because if you go too glitzy, it may actually get caught in your hair, which isn't fun on the stage. Jewelry can include earrings, necklaces and all the added bling that makes you look superbly presented. Don't go for really tacky jewelry because it doesn't look classy and won't get much attention from the judges. They want their winners to look super classy so the better job you can do of presenting yourself in this way, the more likely you are to catch the judge's eyes.

Heels. There are many competitions that will want you to wear clear heels. If the competition does not specify this then you may want to go with heels that match your suit. You should have bought them by the fifth week of training by the time the competition comes you should be very familiar with them. The way your wear your heels can really make or break your chances in the contest, so take it seriously that you do need to practice and practice again, or you will make mistakes in front of the judges. There are various styles of heel and you need to conform to the rules on heel size and color. Remember, there is the possibility that you are able to walk in shoes that are strapless, but this needs to be tried and tested in the shop. Straps do give your ankle more support and it's vital to choose the right shoes for you. If you do go strapless, it's a lot of strain on your feet, and you need to be sure that you are comfortable with that. You also need your feet to look beautiful, so do use creams on your heels so that you don't have dried skin.

Hair. Make sure to have made your hair appointment weeks in advance. This appointment will take place on the day of the competition so you need the salon to be near the location of the competition. Remember that hair accessories are not allowed. It's useful to have a dry run with your hair styling. The reason for this is that the style they produce on the day may not be exactly what you had in mind. If you have already had it styled a week beforehand you can talk through any different things that you want to with the stylist in advance, so there will be no problems on the day.

The Final Week. During this time you will be working on all the finishing touches. Your training is almost over, with just a few workouts left. Get your nails done so that they can look their best for the competition. Also you need to get bikini wax done and exfoliate. A few days before the competition make sure to do a whole body shave. Make sure you have all your supplies packed and ready to go.

What you can expect at the show. You will probably arrive at location the day before the competition and stay at a hotel. You will receive your spray tan by the people that are running the show. You will go into a spray tent to receive your deep tan. After this you are going to have to wear clothing that is old until the competition so that the spray tan won't bleed onto your good clothes. This is the price you will have to pay to experience your bikini competition. If you already have a good quality tan, then this will enhance it. Don't worry about it being too deep because on stage, with all the lights, it won't be as deep as you think.

The morning of the show you will have meetings with the competition organizers. They will give you the rundown on how the competition is going to run. After you have finished with the meetings, you will go and get your hair and makeup done ready for the contest. It's best to have a hairdresser and makeup artist that is accustomed to competitions, because they will know that there will be a bit of waiting around before they can do their work. Then once you have finished this you are just going to have to wait until the show or competition begins. You want to try and stay focused on getting into your competition mode shortly before the contest begins so that you are prepared and ready to strut your stuff when they call your name!

Conclusion

It seems like a lot of fuss and preparation for something that is over so quickly, but it can make a difference to your career. If you are thinking in terms of a long- term career, then the investment will have been worth it.

If you start to do the competition circuit, you will get more confidence and will be able to prepare yourself both physically and mentally because you will know what it's all about. In the meantime, it is hoped that this book will have helped you prepare initially for your first contest.

You will also get to know a lot of people during the contest circuit and will be making friends along the way. Expect a little jealousy in some directions. Some people take their contests very seriously indeed and may try to put you down or try to break your confidence. However, generally other contestants are pleasant to one another and there is a great sense of camaraderie between them. This is the best way to be, because judges do pick up on selfish attitude and on the contest day, it's time to drop the attitude and simply enjoy the contest.

Learn from your mistakes. Learn all the time about how to improve your presentation and you will grow as a contestant and enjoy some of the rewards that come to everyone that competes, rather than just the winners!

Will You Review My Book?

Thank you again for purchasing this book!

I hope this book was able to help you to gather some tips and suggestions that will help you in preparing yourself for your bikini competition.

The next step is to start looking around for a suitable coach that will help you to reach your goals so that you may enter the bikini competition that you have your heart set on.

I hope you liked this book and that you will get as much pleasure from reading it as I've gotten from writing it; it really was a labor of love. I'd like to ask you for a favor, would you be kind enough to leave a review for this book on Amazon? It'd be greatly appreciated!

Thank you and good luck!

Other Recommendations

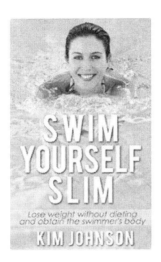

Swim Yourself Slim: Lose Weight Without Dieting and Obtain the Swimmer's Body

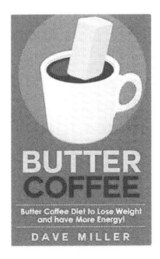

Butter Coffee: Butter Coffee Diet To Lose Weight And Have More Energy

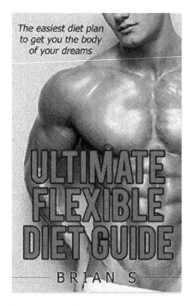

Flexible Dieting: The Easiest Diet Plan To Get You The Body Of Your Dreams

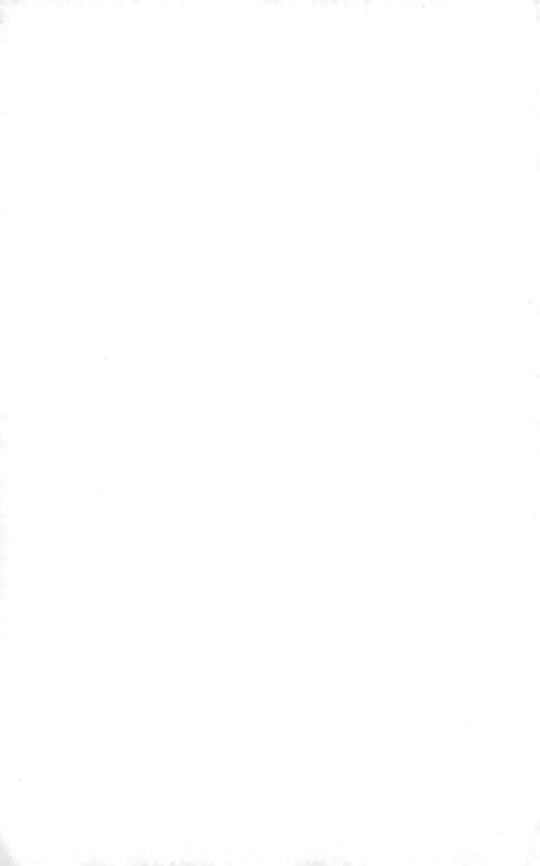

Made in the USA
Lexington, KY
20 November 2016